MW01172229

The Health Benefits of Wild Pine Pollen

Master Builder of Strength and Power

Dr. CASS INGRAM

Knowledge House Publishers

Contents

Chapter 1

Introduction

There are profound substances in nature which are of immense value to human health. They are so powerful in their functions that they are virtually drug-like, that is they offer potent chemicals that have definite effects. Able to reverse many of the conditions which afflict humankind these substances are especially active against age-related degenerative disease. These are the medicines of the pine tree, God's special, protective gifts to this human race. They are specific for blocking and reversing human breakdown. Moreover, synthetically, these natural medicines cannot even be remotely duplicated. In other words, nothing in the sterile, chemical pharmacy can match the power and versatility of tree medicines. The so-called Fountain of Youth was always right before us, and no one ever realized it, at least no one in modern times.

Yet, could pine be that health-giving, as described? It undeservedly has a bad reputation with people, for instance, belittling naturalists, like Ewell Gibbons, for supposedly eating bark or pine cones. This is also because of allergies related to airborne exposure, the high pollen counts that cause so much misery and angst. Yet, both the pollen and bark are emergency foods that were eaten by the primitives without issue. This would have to be so. After all, this substance has the immense potency to incite the growth and development of a powerful tree that lives far beyond the human lifespan. Further, the needles have that special capacity of spreading the pollen, while upholding and maintaining the tree substance. The sap runs through the needle tips, providing nourishment and healing substance. It may be safely harvested from the trunk.

Pollen: superfood of nature

Pine pollen has been recently popularized as a superfood. Yet, when most health enthusiasts think of pollen, it is the type collected by bees. This protein- and nutrient-rich complex is for them a major food source. It typically arises from flowers and herbs, though crops may also represent a source. Pine pollen is a specialized source. Almost drug-like in its actions it could at the minimum serve as a major food source for humans, just as it does for bees. In this respect it could even be an aid in solving world hunger.

Yet, pine pollen is most infamous because of its therapeutic actions. There is much historical precedence for this. Consider the Chinese use, which is extensive. The various applications included a wide array of conditions that confirms that this is one of the most sophisticated, potent natural medicines ever to be discovered in those early centuries. These uses include easing of fatigue, reduction of rheumatic pain, reduction in muscle soreness and pain, enhancement of skin health, improved neurological function, toning of the intestinal tract as well as stomach, increased intestinal cell wall health, strengthening of the heart, elimination of prostate disorders, enhanced mental health, increased muscular strength, and weight reduction. It was also observed that pine, in general, was the means of toning and strengthening the immune system. This is an impressive list, and this was all discovered prior to any modern research on its properties. Chinese practitioners were unaware of the mechanism, but these benefits were arguably the result of its high density of amino acids and endocrine-balancing substances.

Yet, let us evaluate the basics using bees as the example. For them pollen, along with honey, is the sustaining substance. It acts as a natural multiple vitamin-mineral supplement, while also providing the high amounts of amino acids and fatty acids necessary for their existence. Plus, it has the novel property of being dense in substances necessary for survival and longevity: polyphenols, flavonoids, regenerative enzymes, and pigments. This is sufficiently nourishing for royalty, that is the queen bee. Laying up to 3000 eggs per day there is only one reason she could be such a powerhouse of production. It is her ultimate nutrient source, which is pollen. It is converted by the other bees into royal jelly, her sole food. This can only serve the function of sustaining this royal creature mainly because of the great amount of proteins and lipids present but also as a result of the rare-to-find steroid content. Additionally, it provides unknown or secretive factors that defy all attempts at synthesis or isolation. These factors may be just as crucial as all that is known by science.

As a health food plant pollen became popular in the 1960s and 1970s, commonly sold in health food stores. Today, it can still be found, where it is recommended for added strength, allergy reduction, immune resistance, and increased nutritional value. Many people just take it, because it is "good for them' and add it to cereal or oatmeal.

During 1970s it was discovered that certain athletes in various countries, notably in eastern Europe and Russia, relied upon it for their exceptional performance. This was true of a number of Olympic athletes, who resoundingly defeated the Americans. It was also found that in village peoples of Russia and Ukraine longevity was linked to the routine intake of a special mixture of pollen in raw honey. It proved to be a complete food that could sustain them on its own and was easy to digest as well as assimilate. This is particularly true of elderly people with compromised digestion and absorption. Since primitive times people in such regions harvested the pollen, especially from trees, as a survival food source.

For honeybees it is truly immensely valuable. In fact, even for humans it may be regarded as the completely perfect whole food, with one group of researchers calling it the "world's best food" source. Let us consider this nutritionally impressive plant source; carbohydrates, proteins, lipids, fatty acids, steroid hormones, polyphenols, carotenoids, vitamins, and minerals all in one? Because of this density, it is the superior nutritional source to aid all cells and organs. No other food has such variety of diversity and richness for bodily needs. The fact is, it is a great powerhouse for all that could disturb the human body. This is especially true of hormonal disorders. After all, for the queen bee in the form of steroid-rich royal jelly it is that specialized food that vitalizes her, which strengthens the various organ systems: immune, digestive, endocrine, dermatological, and eliminative. This is so she can continue to function to feats of the unfathomable, making her a hundred-fold or more, stronger than any in her colony. It is the steroid hormones in this pollen-based food that leads to her metamorphosis. These substances, which are essentially chemical messengers, work on her genes. These factors are found in the black seed oil specialized pine pollen drops and honey-pollen mix.

Chapter 2

Everyone Benefits

N o doubt, with all its components the pine tree is an enormous blessing for humankind. Whether the needles, pollen, cones, sap (that is resin) or bark, truly, pine is a food and medicine for all people and at every age. The nutritional profile of the needles and pollen alone proves that. The sexual dust is a hormone source, which is rare in the plant kingdom. The fact that it contains testosterone doesn't exclude women, as they need it, too. The hormones are in micro-doses, just like the body makes them. So, that's why all people benefit. Plus, as a result of the plethora of active ingredients pine pollen possesses significant biological activity in various arenas, much of it already indicated by the Chinese use. Of major importance is the fact that this pollen offers antioxidant, antibacterial, antiviral, hepato-protective, and anti-cancer actions, all in one. It has also been demonstrated to provide significant cardio-protective effects, which is crucial. Yet, so do the needles and the resin.

The needles are dense in a variety of nutrients, which are concentrated in them from the flowing sap. These nutrients include vitamin C, of which it is five-times richer than lemons, vitamin A as beta carotene, and also trace minerals. The needles are a natural remedy for the majority of human diseases. In a tincture or tea these needles help alleviate congestion and other respiratory ailments. There are decongestant, disinfectant, and wound healing properties in this tree growth. The needles can be used like applewood in fires to smoke meats or chicken, adding a hint of pine flavor. Or, put them beneath fish while cooking or chop finely, adding to marinades or brine-based preserved foods. For the pollen the greatest domain is the endocrine system.

This is the organ system that controls much of human existence, including internal, vital forces: the ones required for survival. The density in steroids, much needed by the hormonal system, in fact, virtually every gland, cannot be overestimated. This largely explains its immense powers for aiding male endocrine disorders, including impotence and prostatitic conditions. As a rule, so-called benign prostatic hypertrophy, chronic prostatitis, early prostate cancer, erectile dysfunction, and post-menopausal syndrome in women all succumb to its medicinal capacities. No other natural complex can offer this potency for such a wide range of endocrine disorders. With time, the body becomes deficient in these endocrine substances. Pine pollen replenishes them in a major way, positively influencing health in all instances.

Complete food

For all bodily systems nothing could be more nourishing and complete than pine. Mainly the needles and the pollen this includes the full gamut of cellular systems and internal organs. With pollen's 18 different amino acids it contains all that the body needs to sustain itself plus far more, that is various nutraceuticals with medicinal properties. Offering more complete protein than meat and eggs this is the type of protein and amino acid components that are ideally consumed raw. In that state these substances are readily utilized and absorbed.

There is another critical issue. Like royal jelly, pine pollen contains substances unknown by human investigation. The same is true of the needles and the resin. They are too sophisticated and complex for the human scientific mind to determine its full array of components. Even so, it is established, as mentioned, as a primary source of carbohydrates, protein, amino acids, lipids, vitamins, and minerals, along with polyphenols, flavonoids, carotenoids, and pigments.

It is best is to combine the needles with the resin and pollen to gain complete efficacy from its powers. All these have considerable positive effects on human health. Only rarely does a food contain this full complement of medicinal aids. This makes extracts of pine ideal for use in the diets of all people, including children, adults, and the elderly. This is particularly true of those who suffer from vitamin and mineral deficiency as well as the lack of protein and amino acids. Other nutritional components of intense value include its density of carotenoids, which can be considerable. These carotenoids include lutein, beta carotene, and beta crytoxanthin. There is also its rich supply of essential fatty acids, phospholipids, phytosterols, flavonoids, waxes, fiber, aromatic compounds, and resins, plus don't forget the substances unknown. Emulsification in black seed oil, when possible, aids in the utilization and absorption of the fat-soluble compounds, including the phytosterols, essential fatty acids, fat miscible vitamins, and phospholipids.

Did primitive man rely upon it?

In particular, pine pollen is naturally sweet. It is also satisfying and filling. Surely, in pre-history this was well-understood. Yet, what happened during primitive times can only be imagined. Otzi the Ice Man had pine pollen in his digestive tract. Did he consume it to sustain him on his arderous mountainous journey and his fight against the elements? Some claim he merely inhaled it through his mouth. Even so, walking up and down the Alps is no easy feat. Perhaps, the pine pollen gave him the power and energy to do so. Plus, what else could he find to eat at those lofty elevations? It would have been a sustaining wild food that could easily be harvested. Most likely, he was eating it for this purpose. He likely also brewed the needles as tea.

Evergreens: as food and medicine

While it is little known evergreens are, and were, historically, a source of both food and medicine. Since ancient times components of these plants have been relied upon for their sustaining and nutritional offerings. Even the cones of pine and spruce were utilized for food and tea. The berries of juniper were a foodstuff, boiled down into a syrup or added to food. The pollen was one of the easiest sources to harvest and use. Of all evergreens only the pine makes large amounts of it. During the season so much can be produced that it can cover the forest floor. The pollen is the male part, while the ovaries or seeds are found in the cone. The wind blows it from tree-to-tree and all about, so it can fertilize the female parts. With proper timing it can be harvested from pine forests in considerable amounts: without harming the forest structure. It is singlehandedly the best hormone source in wild nature. While the bark, needles, and cones are health-giving, they lack the intense density of steroid hormones found it.

Every year, millions of tons of this golden dust are distributed all over the globe. After leaving the tree rapidly it degenerates. A rainy day causes it to rot and mold, its steroids lost forever. Yet, is there a way to preserve it, so all people will benefit? In springtime pines offer "furry" catkins, which are small protuberances among the needles found nearly at the end of each branch. This usually forms the base for pine nuts and cones. These catkins can be clipped off and consumed raw. With pine needles add these medicinal aids to soups or for fish and meat dishes, especially wild sources. The catkins, along with the needles, are useful throughout the year as a source of tea. Since they are highly concentrated, only a few are necessary for brewing a satisfying cup of tea. The tea available as Purely Wild Pine tea contains the catkins with the needles, largely from white pines.

While few people will harvest pinecones, they are edible. For example, a pinecone can be boiled in soups to add nutrition and flavor. It should be kept in mind that in the wild, a number of wild squirrels virtually subsist on them, typically in the fresh, green state. The inner bark of pine was commonly used as food by Native Americans and early colonists. For the taste-initiated, the inner bark can be stripped, dried and ground to a flour that serves as a nutritious additive to baked goods and other dishes.

Yet, this should be done with caution so not to destroy the tree. As well, only trees far away from heavy pollution should be utilized, certainly not those next to busy highways.

The need for raw honey with pine pollen: mycotoxins and more

The mycotoxins in pine pollen can be considerable. So can bacteria. This is particularly true if it is dried inadequately. There may also be naturally occurring allergens, pyrrolizidine alkaloids, and other unknown toxins. Wild oregano neutralizes these, rendering any mold non-toxic, while also neutralizing allergens. For a specific group of consumers allergic reactions can occur if they are sensitive to pollen. As is well-published, pollen-related food allergy reactions are relatively common. After ingestion, there can be scratchy throat, shortness of breath, swollen tongue, swollen throat, and swelling of the lips as well as asthma-like attacks. Usually, this resolves within 30 minutes. Cooking and heat-drying typically eliminate this.

Is there a way to achieve this without processing or heating? This is one of the key reasons for the addition of raw honey and black seed oil. These virtually eliminate the pollen's allergic reactivity, and they also act as a powerful antihistamine. For instance, black seed oil and raw honey reduce the incidence of hives, itchiness, and anaphylactic shock, which is often manifested by severe oral swelling. Further, as indicated, spice oils allow the pollen to be kept in a raw state. Mycotoxins are not a natural component. This is a result of moldiness which cannot occur unless the pollen was handled inadequately.

Through this, these components can stay fresh despite being exposed to air. Otherwise, the nutrients, especially the vitamins and polyphenols, are readily lost merely over time or improper storage. Always look for pine pollen containing wild oregano oil, either in a liquid or powder phase.

There must be a preservative process. Most purveyors rely upon alcohol, which obviously is less than desirable. In particular, this substance denatures the amino acids, so as therapeutic aids these are lost.

Black seed oil and raw honey are novel additions. It is well- established that microbes thrive on pollen. Bee-collected types typically contain high levels of moisture, which is conducive to the rapid growth of microbial agents. Plus, this facilitates various chemical and enzymatic reactions that are harmful to the end- product. Of note, the background moisture content may be as high as 30%. This is a danger zone, leading to mold and bacterial overload. To prevent this all pollen must be thoroughly dried. Yet, in many instances even this is not enough. What is more the addition of honey is highly protective. Otherwise, with raw pollen spoilage will inevitably occur. The exception would be if it is frozen after purchase or possibly freeze-dried. Yet, these have the untoward effects of destroying the enzymes. Other methods, such as the soaking in alcohol or the application of heat, including hot- air drying, also lead to destructive effects, including loss of the enzymes. As well, both hot air-drying and freeze-drying, also known as lyophilization, lead to the significant loss of proteins and amino acids. If the temperature is increased to above 50 degrees Celsius, the losses may be major at nearly 50%. In contrast, immersion in honey or black seed acts as a preservative and leads to retention of virtually the full complement of these nutrients. Essentially, heat and alcohol dimmish the medical capacities of this substance even as much as 70% compared to the raw. Any cleaning or purification leads to a depletion in nutritional value. The crude grind with its aromatic pine-source compounds retailed helps preserve the content of vitamins especially, including C, E, beta carotene, and the B complex, which may decline significantly. In refined pollen losses of beta carotene alone may reach nearly 80% within a year. If it is stored in a freezer, this reduces the depletion.

Honey also acts as a storage vehicle, and this is what occurs in nature. This may be partly because it halts all enzymatic reactions. Honey-bee pollen combinations are known to possess measurable anti-inflammatory powers and have shown strong antioxidant capacities in lab tests. The spices, though, are the top antioxidants known. Thus, the combination of honey, wild oregano, and pine pollen is ideal. Another medium is to add the raw pollen to yogurt. Letting it sit for a day or two increases the nutritional value and digestibility as well as the antioxidant capacity, noted in part by an increase in polyphenol content. There is a superior taste and overall culinary experience with this combination than the pollen alone. No doubt, adding raw honey would be ideal to this nutritious mix. The pollen and honey greatly add to the viability of healthy bacterial cultures in fermented milk beverages, including yogurt, probiotic milk, and kefir. The crude grind aids this as well by providing a plethora of soluble fiber. The probiotic bacteria flourish on this to the aid of intestinal function. Adding it in the form of the raw honey mix to smoothies or yogurt greatly aids intestinal function and may help resolve constipation.

Chapter 3

Plant Hormones and Human Health

The hormones from certain plants can prove invaluable for human health. These plant hormones are those found in ashwagandha, andrographis extract, saw palmetto, pumpkin (actually its seeds), black seed, wild chaga, fresh sprouts, wheat grass, and pollen. Here, it should be kept in mind that it is rather rare in the plant kingdom to find these steroid-based hormones in density. Even so, plant sterols, that is phytosterols, have been touted for decades for their health benefits. They represent a critical array of natural substances that have numerous biological functions in plants. Yet, this can be co-opted for humans, for instance, dietary phytosterols are able to lower levels of serum cholesterol via the inhibition of its absorption and the compensatory stimulation of its synthesis. Yet, the major new finding is that they may also act as precursors for the internal synthesis of animal hormones and other steroid molecules. Even more crucial is the fact that they act as the actual hormonal agents themselves, mimicking what is produced in the body. These hormone-like components are found in every part of pine - the resin, needles, bark, and pollen.

As in animals, steroids are natural and essential components of plants, where they are act as chemical messengers for cell-to-cell communication. This is required for the regulation of growth and also early sexual development. Therefore, it is obvious that vital, growing plants, the bigger the better, are dense in these steroidal substances. The sexual parts, like the flowers and the pollen, are highest in density.

Pollen from pines contains a higher percentage of testosterone and other androgens than virtually any other source, as would be expected from such a powerful creation. These compounds are also known as brassinosteroids, which are exceptionally specialized as the tree's ultimate signaling molecules. All pine trees contain them. In one Greek study a high content of androsteroids was found in the wild-growing species Pinus nigra and Pinus heldreichii. Yet, this was only realized since the 2000s. Pinus nigra or black pine was found to contain epitestosterone and a number of androsterones. Never before studied Pinus heldreichii has these steroids at a much higher content. Even higher is the powerful tree Pinus brutia, or Mediterranean red pine. It contains the highly active steroid molecules, testosterone, androsterone, estrogen, among numerous others. This is the type of pine pollen used in the high-grade supplements mentioned in this book.

No doubt, there is a negative connotation with these substances. This is particularly in relation to cell growth or cancer. People often worry unnecessarily, so it should be stated clearly. None of these hormones have any toxicity and are not a concern in hormone-related diseases, including estrogen-dependent breast cancers or prostate cancers. These naturally- occurring hormones only aid the body and can by no means cause any harm. Existing within the pollen in micro-doses there is no way to accumulate them.

Signaling molecules for energy and stamina

All steroids are signaling molecules. Thus, they are the most potent natural chemicals known. Pine pollen is a dependable means for achieving a boost in energy. It is a sustained one and can last for 24 hours or more. Yet, this occurs without the irritating effects upon the nerves as occurs with the typical caffeinated energy drinks. For instance, there is no way pine pollen or its extracts will overstimulate the body, leading to both ups and downs. It can't, unlike other supplements burn a person out, and by no means can it irritate the adrenal glands, which caffeine does routinely. What it does is the unfathomable, which is to support the energy production within all cells, aid in the power that is needed for exercise routines and enhance athletic endeavors without the slightest risk for overdoing it. The tea, resin drops, crude extract of needles, and the pollen all offer this capacity. Combine them with supplements containing ashwagandha and/or royal jelly for an additive effect.

Large versus small doses

The power in pine pollen is dose dependent. Smaller doses are subtle, supporting the internal functions of the hormone glands. This includes all the main ones, the pituitary, adrenals, thyroid, and gonads. Now, a person can regardless of the circumstances maintain healthy hormone levels.

In contrast, if large doses are taken, then that is when a great increase in strength is likely. A big dose is two or more tablespoons of the pollen-honey mixture, 8 or more capsules, and four or more dropperfuls. This strength effect is a result of the anabolic actions of the plant androgens. This would be especially noticeable in aging persons.

There is never an issue with over-intake of this natural, native medicine. The steroids are highly medicinal and have a lasting effect. So, in some people a minor dosage is all that may be necessary to gain the desired effect. However, it is a natural, wholesome food. Thus, if a higher amount is desired, it is no issue. For instance, an active athlete might consume two or three times the amount of a sedentary person.

Chapter 4

The Tree of Youth

A s has been made abundantly clear the pine tree and its components are a major guard against the aging process. Meanwhile,
they provide relief against the degenerative conditions that result; cardiovascular, digestive, inflammatory, immune, neurological, or otherwise. Consumption causes people to have a more youthful counte-
nance, even appearance, many reporting they feel "20-years younger."
One user reported that his workload greatly went up and he felt he
went "backwards 30- years." In Asia pine is even a staple ingredient
in beauty products, while rarely used in the West. There, whether
taken internally or applied topically, it is well-known to regenerate the
individual. Perhaps, this is why health wise, Asia has the advantage
over the West. They rely upon pine and its extracts, while Western
people do not. People of Western and Northern countries virtually
never take advantage of it.

Why should pine be consumed for youthfulness? It is to provide
much-needed steroid molecules which most people are deficient in as
well as multiple vitamin sources, which the body sorely needs. This is
infinitely superior to the synthetics people typically consume. These
synthetics provide no anti-aging benefit and with their infestation

with petrochemicals and GMOs do more harm than good. Taoist monks have reported that pine needle tea is associated with long and healthy life.

The nutrients in pine components are desperately needed by the body. A partial list of these invaluable nutrient complexes includes the following, found in the densest amounts in the pollen:

- •vitamin A (as beta carotene)
- •vitamin B1, that is thiamine
- •vitamin B2, that is riboflavin
- •niacin, that is vitamin B3
- •vitamin B6, that is pyridoxine
- •folic acid
- •vitamin C
- •vitamins D & E
- •iron
- •potassium
- •calcium
- •magnesium
- •phosphorus
- •zinc
- •selenium
- •manganese

Other nutrients contained, especially in the pollen, include molybdenum, silicon, and sodium. The dust is also dense in fiber, lignins, and that invaluable age-blocking enzyme, superoxide dismutase. While the focus has been on the density of hormonal substances for reviving male health, the nutritional density of this substance clearly is equally important. Since pollen is the seed family it contains all the components needed to bring the new and vital plant into life. A divine creation of immense strength and power this is no small feat with a sturdy, long-lived—and disease- resistant—pine tree. It couldn't happen without the pollen. There is the nutrients list but also some 70 other vital components, including the enzymes which are readily destroyed by processing and alcohol. It should be noted that it contains nucleic acids, also decimated by the ethanol.

While all parts of the pine are high the content of the nutrients in pollen is considerable. For iron, it is some 20-fold higher than spinach, while in beta carotene it is some 30 times richer than carrots. Plus, unlike semi-synthetic vitamin pills or powders these nutrients are in a naturally charged state and are, thus, complete, highly active, and enriched: by the creative power of God Himself, filled with His healing energy. In essential fatty acids it is three times higher than bee pollen, all in a form of easy bioavailability. Of the vitamins listed, it is pantothenic acid which is found in the most dense supply. This nutrient is essential for steroid hormone synthesis.

Weakness reversed

Especially for men there is a real challenge of weakening of the tissues with age. This is related to the decline of testosterone and similar hormones. There is a corresponding decline in muscle mass. This is a disaster. The heart itself is a muscle. With the age- related drop of steroid hormones its size and pumping power is diminished, increasing the risks for heart attacks and strokes. The skeletal muscles suffer atrophy, especially if the lack is extreme. In fact, a loss of such mass is a major consequence of the deficit. The person becomes physically incapacitated. There is an obvious reduction in the thickness of the muscles, especially in the buttocks and thighs. Such tissues of the back and neck might also diminish. As a result, elderly people might develop a shuffling gate and stooped posture. Through its naturally occurring hormone density pine pollen could help reverse this, often rapidly so, its hormones being powerful enough to re-institute muscular density. Its intake may be associated with a noticeable increase in the size of the muscular tissues, especially in the arms and thighs.

Because of this loss, the desire for exercise is lessened. This is an additive crisis, further contributing to the decline. With the naturally occurring steroids, as found in pine but also royal jelly. and ashwagandha, there is a much-desired increase in muscular strength and possibly density, restoring the desire for physical activity and exercise. The person in such a weakened condition should use the tea, resin drops, crude extract, and pollen for re- building purposes. These natural medicines are particularly ideal for those who have suffered muscle loss and weight loss and for them to use the pine to rebuild the body.

Boosting your steroid intake

Pine pollen is the easy way to do this, either as drops, capsules, or pulverized powder. Yet, there are numerous other means to achieve this. The consumption of animal food is a must, which has the greatest density. Other than avocadoes there is little-to-no density in fruit, and vegetables lack them entirely. However, the reproductive parts of grains, the germ and bran, are a good source. Even more dense are milk, yogurt, cheese, and eggs. Fatty fish is a significant source, as is seafood. Therefore, a vegan diet is a catastrophe for steroid and, therefore, hormone intake. Vegans may become weakened just from this deficiency. This could be corrected through the intake of pine pollen, the richest vegetarian source, and also the resin drops and needle tea.

The pollen has special attributes. Plants must fertilize themselves. This requires the presence of hormones. The germinal parts are high, though in micro-doses, with androgens, testosterone, estrogens, progesterone, and various other sex hormones. These hormones regulate the ability of the plants and animals to 'morph' or become altered into another creation, known appropriately as morphogenesis or metamorphosis. Even to change the sex of the living entity is possible. This is true of the most primitive organisms, all the way up. It is a neglected area that people can through various plant and animal sources, as well as herbal ones, 'eat' their hormones. The diet recommended here is rich in the sources of natural hormones, which is one rich in fats as well as animal foods.

Regarding their formation in cells of trees, cholesterol-like molecules are the basis, formed via a special metabolic pathway known as MVA. This is how estrogen and testosterone are formed in such higher plants. It is complex, and no drug or GMO can duplicate it. Rather, they greatly interfere with it. The MVA system operates in the cytosol of plant cells. In the case of phytosterols these are made up of acetic acid molecular units. To produce them is an intensive process requiring an astounding 30 enzymatic steps, all this happening along the plant cell membranes. These phytosterols are starting points for the biosynthesis of the plant steroid signaling molecules, phytoecdysteroids, and the plant steroid hormones brassinosteroids, as well as progesterone, testosterone and its derivatives.

Corticosteroids are a big deal

Foods or herbs that are a dense source of corticosteroids, that is cortisone-like agents, are of immense value for human health. These are one of the most commonly prescribed drug categories, for instance, cortisone, dexamethasone, and Prednisone. To find natural sources that contain this is rare. Pine pollen is one such source.

For the villagers pine is a major medicine of wide utility. In primitive parts of the Mediterranean the village people have utilized the pine tree for centuries. Making use of all parts there are dozens of reports for Pinus species acting as cures for various diseases. These diseases include disorders of the skin, the digestive system, and as an agent of wound healing. Much lesser was the reliance for kidney and bladder conditions, but the needle tea and resin drops would be good for this. There was a fair amount of ethnic use for pain relief purposes, with according to a Turkish study 'other' categories included as an "antimicrobial, antiseptic, aphrodisiac, anthelmintic, fatigue, fracture, topical use as hygienic for teeth, inflammatory diseases, internal disease, lactagogue or milk production," and as a sedative. While no claims are made for any company or product line these are the historical use, which must be given significant consideration.

Attacking the collapse syndrome

Heart attacks and the onset of circulatory disease including stroke, are rare in youth. So is the development of dementia. manifested by Alzheimer's disease. With time, the heart muscle itself becomes weakened. So do the arteries. Without testosterone, the heart muscle loses muscle mass, which can be replaced by mere connective tissue. A sudden heart attack or death can occur, and it was all because of testosterone lack. A person must fight back against this negative, destructive trend. Pine is precisely the tool to do so. It provides the hormonal agents necessary to block this breakdown and to reverse any degenerative trends. Use it also to treat these conditions, the black seed oil-fortified sublingual drops being especially potent. Hypertension is part of this breakdown. Use the pine pollen drops, about 20 drops twice daily, to combat this. Also, it in powder and/or capsules. Consume, as well, the tea and wild resin. Because of the lack of testosterone, muscles in the arteries and heart weaken over time. No one can afford to suffer this. Pine is the top herbal supplement for reversing this trend.

An inflammation attacker

Wherever there is inflammation pine attacks this. In part, this is because it is a dense source of both anti-inflammatory nutrients and steroid compounds. In one study arthritis was artificially induced in test animals. The arthritis was "markedly suppressed," as was the swelling, in the pine pollen groups. The study suggested that this natural food is effective for arthritis or any other inflammatory joint disease, including rheumatoid cases. In particular, the pollen eliminated inflammatory forms of collagen. Yet another investigation, this time by Korean authors, found that the pollen is such a potent antioxidant that it aids in the reversal of chronic inflammatory disorders. In Yugoslavia it was found that perhaps a mechanism for the anti-arthritic effect is it is a good source of vitamin D and its metabolites. Vegetable sources of these nutrients are rare.

Is aging a hormone decline syndrome?

It is well-established that in aging there is a decline in the body's hormone production. This is true of all glands, including the pituitary, thymus, ovaries, testes, adrenals, and thyroid. All the various steroids impact growth and reproduction as well as the prevention of aberrant growths, like tumor cells. When hormonal levels decline or are disrupted, there is a major change in a human's characteristics. Women lose their womanhood, and men lose their manhood. The body fully breaks down and all youthfulness is lost. Now, there is the power of pine pollen. Suddenly, the body is revived. Both men and women gain much of their original characteristics, because now, there are proper hormone levels in the blood. These new-found steroids act on the genes, controlling them and preventing age-related breakdown.

A study by Chinese investigators delineates this. In a mouse study as a model for artificial aging pine pollen was found to retard this process and was held to potentially halt age-related diseases in humans. This was through acting directly on the genes which facilitate this decline. These same components act on the genetic material that impacts inflammation. In an investigation published in Phytotherapy

Research it was held beneficial for degeneration-related inflammation, once again by influencing the genes. Put simply, pine pollen calms the body down, so it doesn't react so violently to stress or age-related toxicities. This partly involves its action against free radicals, that is toxic forms of oxygen, which are associated with heart disease, stroke, hypertension, diabetes, liver disorders, arthritis, cancer, and far more.

Changing your life

Nothing is more powerful than the hormones. In a study in the 1930s a man who had his testicles removed underwent a surgery where an ovary was sewn into his body. His whole body changed, and he turned into a functioning woman with breasts and female- like shape and genitalia. Both estrogen and testosterone, as well as the androgens, have this capacity. For instance, the application of estrogen can dramatically impact sex determination of flowers of plants with both male and female flowers. The hormones can prove so powerful that they can change the sex of the plant. In contrast, other nutraceuticals, like vitamins, minerals, amino acids, polyphenols, flavonoids, and essential fatty acids, are incapable of doing so. A person should consume the pollen, needle tea, and resin drops to gain these benefits.

Waking up earlier will be a side-effect

Mediterranean-sourced pine from wild trees has a special power to be reckoned with. It makes the individual noticeably more productive. One way it does so is that it causes increased capacity for sound sleep. This is deep REM sleep that results from its ingestion. There is a natural decline of cortisol that occurs, but not too low. As a result. the individual has a desire to sleep at a reasonable time. Often, a bit more can be taken at night to stabilize the cortisol levels further. If this is not done, the blood sugar may fluctuate, leading to sleeplessness. Yet, then, it gives the body such internal strength that it requires less sleep.

This can be significant, and a person may wake up one to three hours early, though not in a groggy state. Instead, there will be full wakefulness and a desire to work. So, the individual will be more productive and able to accomplish feats previously impossible. Sleep can be a waste of time, and this will allow a maximum potential. This is especially valuable for salespersons, businesspersons, preachers, and writers or authors. Count on it. Mediterranean pine pollen will help you achieve this. So will far- northern white pine needle tea or extract. The same could be expected from white pine, especially the raw resin extract.

Chapter 5

The Testosterone Issue

The term testosterone is derived from testes. It is the male hormone that drives what makes a person masculine. Directly, it is responsible for sexual characteristics, like pubic hair growth, testicular development, and sperm production. The desire and capacity for sex itself is driven by this substance. Like other hormones it acts as a chemical messenger that triggers essential functions in the body, including healthy muscular strength and cardiovascular function. Of note, females also make testosterone, usually in smaller amounts. Testosterone is an androgen that is produced in the testicles, while to a lesser degree in the adrenal glands. Red blood cell synthesis, the development of sound muscular structure, muscular power/strength, proper fat distribution, and the thickening of the bones are also testosterone- dependent.

It is important to note that the brain and pituitary gland control testosterone levels. Once produced, the hormone moves through the blood to carry out its various important functions. High or low levels of testosterone can lead to dysfunction in the parts of the body normally regulated by the hormone. Small amounts of circulating testosterone are converted to estradiol, a form of estrogen. As men age, they often make less testosterone, but they also produce less estradiol as well. This lack of estrogen compounds also has a negative effect, as this compound plays a role in sexual health.

Extremely low testosterone is known as hypogonadism, the prefix meaning low or insufficient. It is associated with predictable consequences or symptoms, which have already largely been mentioned but here is the list for extreme cases:

•low testosterone, or hypogonadism, he may experience:

•reduced sex drive

•low sperm count

•weakened heart muscle

•erectile dysfunction

•swollen breast tissue

Eventually, this condition may manifest with extreme male pattern baldness and generalized loss of body hair. Muscular mass is lost, and there is a corresponding reduction in strength. The body may become malformed with increased body fat, and the abdomen often becomes rotund, a beer-belly appearance. This is true even in those who don't drink.

The hormone is supremely important for nervous system balance. Thus, chronic, persistent deficiency often leads to depression, irritability, anger fits, and mood swings.

Chronic, or ongoing, low testosterone may lead to osteoporosis, mood swings, reduced energy, and testicular atrophy. Yet, people with certain diseases are more vulnerable to the imbalance. This includes diabetes, liver disorders, obesity, kidney disease, opiate addiction, and HIV/AIDS. Infection of the testicles is an obvious factor, as is trauma and genetic factors such as impaired pituitary function, hemochromatosis, and Klinefelter syndrome. The Mediterranean-source pollen and the far-northern white pine needles are ideal for this purpose.

Infertility

There can be no doubt that pine pollen is a major natural, whole food complex for reversing infertility. This is especially true of the male type. One study on the P. brutia species found a major benefit. Sperm were actually lengthened. Sperm glutathione levels also rose significantly. Essentially, it prevented chromatin damage by reducing oxidative stress in addition to reducing mutations in the sperm head. Regardless, it is a hard fact. When testosterone levels are inadequate, men become infertile. This is because testosterone assists the development of mature sperm.

Even though it is a male sex hormone women naturally make it. For them it is needed for sex drive, bone density, and muscle strength. However, an excess of testosterone can also cause them to experience male pattern baldness, male-type hair growth, and infertility. This cannot occur with pine pollen, as it regulates the production.

Chapter 6

Natural Estrogen, Anyone?

Despite this being the male form of fertilizing agent, pine pollen is a good source of female hormones. These hormones include primarily estrogen and progesterone. Plus, these molecules are interchangeable, so that, for instance, testosterone can be readily converted to forms of estrogen, notably estradiol. Thus, there is a value in the pollen for both males and females. Of note, for men there is no harm of consuming vegetable-source estrogens. Nor is there any harm in women. In fact, these are estrogenic substances of divinely sophisticated medicines. As such, they actually block the toxicity of human estrogens, the ones that in some circumstances provoke cancer development.

Some plant estrogens, though, are not healthy. The best example are those from soy, especially from the genetically engineered varieties. These estrogens are poisonous and are fully unfit for human consumption. Pine estrogens, in contrast, do not cause any such untoward effects.

What pine pollen steroids do is interfere with the metabolism of the more toxic forms. This is via their influence on various metabolic pathways, including the mevalonate one that produces the isoprenoids. These molecules are necessary to vital cellular functions which range from growth control to cholesterol synthesis. The system is directly influenced by pine pollen to block excessive cellular growth, which may lead to cancer. In addition, it will aid in maintaining steady function of the heart muscle. Think of it as a normalizer to prevent toxic forms of testosterone or estrogen from agitating the cells. For this reason, regular consumption is advisable.

The molecules that enter this pathway are essential for cellular growth. When it is uncontrolled, pathology results. It is being researched heavily in the fields of oncology, autoimmune disorders, atherosclerosis, and neurological disease.

When the pine pollen is consumed, the astonishing occurs. There is an immediate boost in energy. This is true both crude powder as well as the sublingual emulsified drops. This is largely a result of the steroid content, but it may also be due to the rich supply of amino acids and vitamins. It is the most dependable energy-boosting agent possible, far more so than the typical highly caffeinated energy drinks. It is also more potent than the typically considered energy boosters, including ashwagandha and ginseng.

When men pass their 40s, they are prone to a male menopausal syndrome. Known as adropause, this is represented by a decline in the synthesis of androgenic hormones, particularly testosterone. Libido is obviously affected, as is internal strength and energy. There is an increased risk for moodiness and depression, while there is also increased muscular fatigue.

The amino acid factor

The animo acids in pine pollen are one of its major components. These biologically critical substances are directly utilized by the body. For instance, consider its phenylalanine content in which it is rich. This amino acid is associated with the release of neurotransmitters in the brain. Thus, it is a common supplement for pain syndromes and also as an antidepressant. It is this amino acid which stimulates dopamine levels in the brain, as it is a precursor for L-dopa. Moreover, L-dopa has been known to be effective in treating the inability in woman to have orgasms. Pine pollen also contains arginine, which improves fertility in women and men, as well as, increases growth hormone release.

All people could use more amino acids, especially in the raw state. Unless a person is eating raw cheese, milk, or eggs this is difficult to achieve. Through unprocessed pine pollen, the person can consume up to 20 different raw amino acids and get the full benefits they offer. Pine pollen has up to 10 times the protein content of red meat or eggs, which means it is perhaps the most dense source of this nutrient known.

The gut factor

Pine pollen is incredibly valuable for gut health. This is especially true of the type which is emulsified in black seed oil, although all truly raw material is invaluable. A study was done by Chinese investigators to determine the influence of this wild plant material on the gut microecology of rats. It was found that the pine pollen protected gut flora from the influence of stress and forced activity, which inevitably leads to a decline. The pollen effectively prevented noxious bacteria from over-populating the tissue. The conclusion was that the "Feeding the rats pine pollen can efficiently alleviate the gut microecological disturbance caused by the chronic stresses..."

In daily use this wild natural medicine dramatically boosts gut health. Elimination is facilitated, the food being more well- digested. Constipation is readily alleviated by the pine pollen prescription.

Do alcohol and pollen mix?

Commonly on the market are found alcohol tinctures of this natural complex. Does this make sense? If anything, it should be in its own matrix, in the pine resin or pine terpene base. Alcohol is foreign to pine pollen and, in fact, destroys its invaluable enzymes, including SOD and catalase. Plus, it oxidizes most of its proteins and amino acids. Far superior to this is to emulsify it in a natural oil base such as black seed oil. Now, the pollen is complete with its enzymes fully intact. In contrast, in ethanolic extracts some 80% of the active ingredients are neutralized or destroyed. Alcohol is harsh, while, in contrast, pine pollen is exceedingly delicate. The two cannot mix to any degree. Avoid all pine pollen alcohol extracts.

Chapter 7

How to Use Pine Pollen

There are several ways to consume this wondrous substance. It can be taken internally as non-alcoholic emulsified drops, as a crude powder to mix in fluids, and as capsules. medicinal tinctures, used as powders mixed in food or drink, or can be used topically by being made into a cream or paste and applied directly to the skin. Topically-applied pine pollen is ideal for the treatment of eczema, diaper rash, psoriasis, dermatitis, or other skin irritations. Alternatively, the drops in black seed oil can be applied as a cosmetic agent. Pine pollen powder is also a valuable aid. Fortified with wild oregano and cinnamon powders this makes a convenient, nutritious addition to water, juice, and smoothies. It can also be dusted into soup or over stir-fry, poultry, casseroles, and steak. Added to yogurt or cottage cheese, it greatly fortifies it, making a meal in itself.

It should be kept in mind that pine pollen has a major protective action. It must be taken just for this purpose. This is versus cellular breakdown, hormonal breakdown, and cancer. In particular, the steroids it contains are active against various carcinomas, particularly breast and prostate. The components work to normalize cancer-vulnerable tissues. For instance, it can significantly reduce the size of an enlarged prostate, while doing the opposite when necessary, increasing its size. In other words, it blocks atrophy if the prostate is too small. With its rich content of biological agents, pine pollen directly interferes with all cancer cell growth and multiplication. This is a crucial capacity, since there are other hormone sources that increase disease risk. This is notably the estrogenic agents that pollute the water supply, and there is a direct correlation between these toxins and the increased incidence of these cancers.

Cracked cell walls—is it necessary?

Many sources claim that pine pollen is difficult to digest. Supposedly, it can't easily be broken down by human digestion. There is no evidence for this. In fact, it is to the contrary. People have been utilizing this natural food-like medicine for centuries. The Chinese, for one, have some 3000 years of usage, claiming great benefits, while never seeking to 'crack' or manipulate the cell walls. There was never an issue of absorption then and no special processing was applied, so there isn't any issue now.

One of the most ancient of all cultures, which has always been medically aware, reveres this natural medicine for thousands of years for good reason. There is obviously a high status for it. Yet, so little of this world despite all its advances knows about it. Certainly, virtually no one realizes that it is a nutrient-dense food. With over 200 bioactive nutrients, vitamins, and minerals in high concentrations, it is one of the most nutritious wild foods available. Of all the world's natural complexes it rates the highest in the capacity to stimulate hormone production, especially testosterone.

Pine pollen is actually a seed. In this regard it contains all the biological substances required of such a natural, sophisticated complex but, in particular, to grow a towering 100-foot tall pine tree that can live for hundreds of years. As such, it contains an incredibly wide spectrum of unique and rare substances that do much the same for the human body as they do for the trees: rapid growth, rejuvenation, powerful, resilient structure, resistance against disease, and exceptional healing capacities. This is so much so that it is widely considered to be the top natural medicine in the world for such properties. Cracked cell walls is of no consequence and amounts to excessive processing. As it is in nature it is ready for consumption. Pine pollen should undergo the least degree of processing possible. As it is it is fully digestible, nothing draconian needs to be done to it. This makes the honey emulsion, where it remains fully unaltered, ideal for human consumption.

Complete cellular rejuvenation, longevity, and more

In the Orient pine pollen is known as a powerful Jing-enhancing herb, which loosely translates to vital essence or life- force. Herbs classified in the Jing realm are typically used in cases of extreme weakness, stress-related burnout, feebleness, incapacitation, gross fatigue, exhaustion, infertility, and sexual disturbances such as erectile dysfunction and low libido. Because of its rich steroid content, it is the ideal natural medicine for whole body revival. Here, it must be kept in mind that it is these compounds which are nuclear activators. There is little if anything else in the body that can do so, that can directly influence the genes. The steroids of pine pollen fine tune the genetic material, leading to the potential for internal vitality or youthfulness. After all, the hormones control the cellular processes. Without them, there is no means of survival. In their absence or deficiency, the body is unable to function, and the person is incapable of coping. All the tissues suffer from the deficit, and consequently the body falters under the pressure.

Pine pollen is naturally spread by the wind, and during the reproductive season of the pine tree. It tends to coat the ground and other nearby plants in testosterone and a number of other hormones that are useful for helping to stimulate growth and reproduction. Clearly, to almighty God pine pollen is special for His creation, while for the majority of humans, it is completely ignored. It is just a yellow, sticky dust, a nuisance, which dirties up the porch or the outside of the car.

Pollen dust for all

Playing with and handling pollen dust might be beneficial beyond imagination. It is clearly God's gift for all people with the trees and their dust being found in virtually all corners of the earth. Despite their being unmistakably towering and magnificent in structure people don't realize it. In suburban and city life no one even in the least degree considers harvesting them. Despite this, it is possible that pine pollen is actually beneficial for the growth of young people during the warmer seasons. Children are typically exposed to the tree's growth-inducers, including testosterones and estrogens, when they are playing outside in the spring and early summer. No doubt, the added hormones, even in micro doses, can help accelerate their growth, as they gain little exposure from any other. No wonder they love playing outside and under the trees or in woods, not tolerating being indoors. People should make a point of getting the children outdoors during pollen season, but make sure and watch for the ticks.

Needle tea to the rescue

Pine needle tea must be made readily available. This is ideally from the American and Canadian white pine, which is the most edible species. Made fresh, it is, as mentioned, a dense source of vitamins C and A. There is also the benefit of the oxygenated terpenes, which give great benefits to the nerves. A cup or two per day helps maintain good health, especially of the nervous system and immune function. There will also be a positive action on the digestive tract and urinary system. The crude extract may prove even more potent and is an option for those who do not drink tea.

The magic of tree resin

The medicine in the pine tree is found in the resin. It is this that gives it life and transports crucial nutrients such as sterols and oxygen, the latter in the form of oxygenated terpenes. This natural medicine is available as drops under the tongue and as a component of an eight-ounce bottle with oregano juice and spruce extract (also rich in oxygen). It can, as well, be found in a cream base with spruce resin for skin cell regeneration. This sticky substance is a major digestive aid, especially for the stomach, and also an antiparasitic agent. Of note, turpentine, made from resin, is an anti- worm agent, though much harsher than the edible resin. To gain the maximum benefits of all these trees has to offer also consume supplements fortified with the resin. Conditions which respond to this include skin disorders, especially psoriasis, stomach ailments, esophageal disorders, intestinal conditions, and worm overload.

Motivation medicine

It is fully established that those with low testosterone are generally impaired. This applies to both physical and mental health problems.

They could in general be depressed. In some cases, this may even be severe. The depression may be all a result of an apathy or lack of motivation, which is not psychological but is, rather, strictly physical. This will all rapidly disappear with Mediterranean pine pollen therapy, especially if it is combined with the needle tea. This is a sun-charged form of pollen that still retains its vital energy, just as it was on the tree. Japanese studies have found that just walking through forests alleviated depression, just from inhalation of micro-doses of pine medicine. Merely from walking in the forest on the beds of needles, they determined, there were benefits to the nervous system.

Chapter 8

Conclusion

The elements of wild pine are among those rare natural complexes that act to revive body function. There is little available that has this power. Through the intake of the various pine components this is a significant way people can feel better. It will be a new experience to consume it, a positive one in all cases. The people of the East know this, ingesting pine regularly with emphasis on the pollen. Yet, all societies must take advantage of it. The fact is pine in all its aspects will make people more productive, vitalizing civilization. Allergy may prove a contraindication. Perhaps, this can be minimized through the oregano oil formulas, where small doses can be tolerated. There is a method for determining this. Using the sublingual drops a tiny amount, like a drop, can be taken under the tongue or rubbed on the skin. If this is tolerated, the dosage may be increased to tolerance. Some people will prove excessively allergic and may not be able to take any dosage. For the rest of the people, it could prove a staple, providing high nutrition, strength, and energy for all. Honey also blocks this allergic tendency. Even so, beware of any pine supplement which undergoes heat treatment or sterilization, as this greatly disrupts the molecular structure of its components. Usually, only a small percentage, like 10%, of its powers will survive.

Certain types of pine are less than ideal. These pine trees are even thought to contain toxins. These types of trees include ponderosa and the pine relatives, yew and cyprus. Actually, any pine tree that is commercially grown or is a desert species is not the health-giving type. Stick with the Mediterranean red pine and also American and Canadian white pine; they have the longest history for human use with no toxicity or irritating effects. In particular, all aspects of white pine are optimal for human use and can be consumed without issue on a daily basis. The moral of the story is to know the source, with North American white pine being ideal, especially for needle tea.

Pine is a weight loss medicine. After all, the needles are skinny-thin. Moreover, the needles contain a thinness hormone. The increase in metabolism from the tea or pollen may be considerable. There is generally an enhancement of body temperature. The skin temperature often goes up noticeably. Just like the trees through this prescription people tolerate the cold better and, in fact, often become oblivious to it.

Because of the micro-hormone content, the entire endocrine system is enhanced. It is in a manner of an impressive degree beyond anything that other herbal supplements could achieve. The thyroid gland functions superiorly, as do the adrenals. With every dose the pituitary receives a much-deserved rest. The gonads are greatly and positively impacted, and the age- weakened ovaries and testes are greatly supported. Hardly any gonadal disorder can withstand its powers, including polycystic ovarian syndrome, PMS, infertility, and impaired libido. All this would be enhanced through the intake of royal jelly and ashwagandha, available as a novel, combined formula.

In men there is a benefit to the prostate, and it becomes far less vulnerable to cancerous degeneration. For tough cases both the sublingual black seed oil drops and the powder or capsules should be taken. Black seed oil itself contains steroidal compounds. The combination is extremely potent for reversing all hormonal disruptions.

So, take advantage of this stupendous natural medicine. Consume it to gain the key benefit of increased stamina. Take it to increase physical strength and athletic skills. Or, just consume it as a tool to ward off disease. Pine pollen is being intensively studied, particularly since 2004.

According to the World Journal of Traditional Chinese Medicine the top arenas of its investigation include as an antioxidant, its liver protection powers, as a means of inhibiting prostate cell overgrowth, that is hyperplasia, for blocking tumor cell formation, for reducing blood sugar, and diminishing excessive blood fats. The main diseases it was found useful in have largely already been mentioned. Yet, an overview is insightful and includes reliable results for bedsores, elevated LDL/total cholesterol, eczema, dermatitis, including diaper rash and cradle cap, high blood pressure, diabetes type II, and high blood pressure. For weight loss an ideal amount is four cups per day, along with the intake of at least one dropperful of pollen drops.

How could any natural medicine be that diverse in its actions? It makes sense, as this is an entire, powerful tree which is highly medicinal. The point is the body is in decline, especially past 55 years of age, and so if it is 'fed' steroids, also in decline, it will begin to thrive. The resin drops, needle tea, and pollen would all be productive in this regard. Plus, the individual needs desperately the nutrients, and it is in a density only seen in this tree medicine. Vigorously use the Mediterranean pine pollen and far-northern white pine needle tea as nutritional supplements, especially for people with poor eating habits and/or a history of hormonal disorders. It doesn't matter. Pine pollen is so rich in nutrients it can work as a true multiple vitamin-mineral treatment, being far superior to any pills or formulas as commonly used. Use it as the preferred whole food multiple vitamin complex. It essentially provides all the body needs, without the synthetics.

So, it is time to relish in all that is pine. Take advantage of this not-so-hidden secret for better health. There are these trees all over the world. They are there for a reason. There are a multitude of forms available. Take advantage of at least the pollen and the tea. If possible, add the crude, raw extract if the needles as an eight-ounce bottle and the resin drops. Select only companies that exclusively harvest the Mediterranean red pine and the delicate Canadian-American white pine. While relying upon these sources the entire pine tree will be in your possession. Plus, like this ubiquitous tree make pine essences a part of your life by consuming its components and gaining the strength of one of the most long-lived and powerful trees known. Use both species to the betterment of health, and always remember there are special attributes to the growths of far-northern forests. The Mediterranean region, when remote, also has a special energy. Take advantage of both of these, and gain that specialized improvement in health that only wild nature can achieve.

Bibliography

Chamawan, P., et al. 2017. Effects of Pine Pollen Extract in Relieving Hot Flushes in Sex Hormone-Deficienct Rats. Thai J. Pharma. 39. Vol. 1.

Graikou, K. and I. Chinou. 2013. Qualitative and quantitative determination of natural testosterone type steroids in pollen from two Greek Pinus species (P. nigra and P. heldreichii). Planta Med. 79 - P128.

Hartmann, M.-A. 1998. Plant sterols and the membrane environment. Trends Plant Sci. 3, 170–175.

Janeczko, A. 2012. The presence and activity of progesterone in the plant kingdom. Steroids. 77: 169–17314.

Kostić, A. Z., et al. (Jan. 2020 online). The Application of Pollen as a Functional Food and Feed Ingredient—The Present and Perspectives. Biomolecules. 10:84.

Lee, K-H., Kim, A-J., and E-M. Choi. 2009. Antioxidant and antiinfammatory activity of pine pollen extract in vitro. Phytotherapy Research. 23:41.

Lindsey, K., Pullen, M.L., and J.F. Topping. 2003. Importance of plant sterols in pattern formation and hormone signalling. Trends Plant Sci. 2003, 8, 521–525.

Moghadasian, M.H. and J.J. Frohlich. 1999. Effects of dietary phy-tosterols on cholesterol metabolism and atherosclerosis: Clinical and experimental evidence. Am. J. Med. 107:588–594.

Payne, A.H.; Hales, D.B. Overview of steroidogenic enzymes in the pathway from cholesterol to active steroid hormones. Endocrin. Rev. 2004, 25, 947–970.

Saden-Krehula, M., Tajic, M., and D. Kolbah. 1979. Sex hormones and corticosteroids in pollen of Pinus nigra. Phytochemistry.

Sláma, K. 1980. Development and metamorphosis in inverte-brates–hormonal control. Gen. Comp. Endocrinol.

Tarkowská, D.; Strnad, M. 2018. Isoprenoid-derived plant sig-naling molecules: Biosynthesis and biological importance. Planta. 247:1051–1066

Taşdemir, Umut., et al. Red pine (Pinus brutia Ten) bark tree ex-tract preserves sperm quality by reducing oxidative stress and prevent-ing chromatin damage.

Thai J Pharmacol. Vol. 39: No. 1,

About Author

Cass Ingram is a nutritional physician who received a B.S. in biology and chemistry from the University of Northern Iowa (1979) and a D.O. from Des Moines Osteopathic College (1984). In the 1980's he started the Arlington Preventive Medical Center in Arlington Heights Illinois, which later became the American Center for Curative Medicine. Ingram was a pioneer in the holistic and preventive medical field. He has written over 25 books on natural healing and has given answers and hope to millions through lectures on thousands of radio and TV shows. His research and writing have led to countless nature based cures and discoveries. Cass Ingram presents hundred's of health tips and insights in his many books on health, nutrition, and disease prevention. He is one of North America's leading pioneers in the field of preventive medicine, with his most famous books *The Cure is in the Cupboard*, *The Cure is in the Forest*, and *Foods that Cure*. He spent his entire life advocating the health benefits and disease fighting properties of wild medicinal foods and spice extracts.

If you found this book beneficial, you would love *Natural Cures From Wild Tree Resin*. For more of Dr. Ingrams books, see purelywild.cassingram.com.

Made in the USA
Columbia, SC
06 January 2025

49320799R00028